Summary

Update: On June 20, 2012, the House of Representatives passed, by voice vote and under suspension of the rules, S. 3187 (EAH), the Food and Drug Administration Safety and Innovation Act, as amended. This bill would reauthorize the FDA prescription drug and medical device user fee programs (which would otherwise expire on September 30, 2012), create new user fee programs for generic and biosimilar drug approvals, and make other revisions to other FDA drug and device approval processes. It reflects bicameral compromise on earlier versions of the bill (S. 3187 [ES], which passed the Senate on May 24, 2012, and H.R. 5651 [EH], which passed the House on May 30, 2012). The following CRS reports provide overview information on FDA's processes for approval and regulation of drugs:

- CRS Report R41983, *How FDA Approves Drugs and Regulates Their Safety and Effectiveness*, by Susan Thaul.

- CRS Report RL33986, *FDA's Authority to Ensure That Drugs Prescribed to Children Are Safe and Effective*, by Susan Thaul.

- CRS Report R42130, *FDA Regulation of Medical Devices*, by Judith A. Johnson.

- CRS Report R42508, *The FDA Medical Device User Fee Program*, by Judith A. Johnson.

(Note: The rest of this report has not been updated since November 10, 2011.)

With the Best Pharmaceuticals for Children Act (BPCA) and the Pediatric Research Equity Act (PREA), Congress authorized the Food and Drug Administration (FDA) to offer drug manufacturers financial and regulatory incentives to test their products for use in children. Congress extended both programs with the FDA Amendments of 2007 (FDAAA) and, because of the programs' sunset date, must act before October 1, 2012, to continue them. This report presents the historical development of BPCA and PREA, their rationale and effect, and FDAAA's impact. The report also discusses pediatric drug issues that remain of concern to some in Congress.

Most prescription drugs have never been the subject of studies specifically designed to test their effects on children. In these circumstances, clinicians, therefore, may prescribe drugs for children that FDA has approved only for adult use; this practice is known as off-label prescribing. Although some clinicians may believe that the safety and effectiveness demonstrated with adults would hold for younger patients, studies show that the bioavailability of drugs—that is, how much gets into a patient's system and is available for use—varies in children for reasons that include a child's maturation and organ development and other factors. The result of such off-label prescribing may be that some children receive ineffective drugs or too much or too little of potentially useful drugs; or that there may be side effects unique to children, including effects on growth and development.

Drug manufacturers are reluctant to test drugs in children because of economic, ethical, legal, and other obstacles. Market forces alone have not provided manufacturers with sufficient incentives to overcome these obstacles. BPCA and PREA represent attempts by Congress to address the need for pediatric testing. FDA had tried unsuccessfully to spur pediatric drug research through administrative action before 1997. With the FDA Modernization Act of 1997 (FDAMA, P.L. 105-115), Congress provided an incentive: if a manufacturer completed pediatric studies that FDA requested, the agency would extend the company's market exclusivity for that product for six months, not approving the sale of another manufacturer's product during that period. In 2002, BPCA (P.L. 107-109) reauthorized this program for five years.

In 1998, to obtain pediatric use information on the drugs that manufacturers were not studying, FDA published the Pediatric Rule, which required manufacturers to submit pediatric testing data at the time of all new drug applications. In 2002, a federal court declared the rule invalid, holding that FDA lacked the statutory authority to promulgate it. Congress gave FDA that authority with PREA (P.L. 108-155). PREA covers drugs and biological products and includes provisions for deferrals, waivers, and the required pediatric assessment of an approved marketed product.

In extending BPCA and PREA in 2007, Congress considered several issues: Why offer a financial incentive to encourage pediatric studies when FDA has the authority to require them? How does the cost of marketing exclusivity—including the higher prices paid by government—compare with the cost of the needed research? What percentage of labeling includes pediatric information because of BPCA and PREA? Do existing laws provide FDA with sufficient authority to encourage pediatric studies and labeling? Is FDA doing enough with its current authority? The 112th Congress will likely consider those questions as well as others: What information do clinicians and consumers need and how could industry and government develop and disseminate it? How can Congress balance positive and negative incentives to manufacturers for developing pediatric information to use in labeling? How could Congress consider cost and benefit when it deals with reauthorizing legislation in 2012?

Contents

Tables

Appendixes

Contacts

Introduction

Update: On June 20, 2012, the House of Representatives passed, by voice vote and under suspension of the rules, S. 3187 (EAH), the Food and Drug Administration Safety and Innovation Act, as amended. This bill would reauthorize the FDA prescription drug and medical device user fee programs (which would otherwise expire on September 30, 2012), create new user fee programs for generic and biosimilar drug approvals, and make other revisions to other FDA drug and device approval processes. It reflects bicameral compromise on earlier versions of the bill (S. 3187 [ES], which passed the Senate on May 24, 2012, and HR 5651 [EH], which passed the House on May 30, 2012). The following CRS reports provide overview information on FDA's processes for approval and regulation of drugs:

- CRS Report R41983, *How FDA Approves Drugs and Regulates Their Safety and Effectiveness*, by Susan Thaul.

- CRS Report RL33986, *FDA's Authority to Ensure That Drugs Prescribed to Children Are Safe and Effective*, by Susan Thaul.

- CRS Report R42130, *FDA Regulation of Medical Devices*, by Judith A. Johnson.

- CRS Report R42508, *The FDA Medical Device User Fee Program*, by Judith A. Johnson.

(Note: The rest of this report has not been updated since November 10, 2011.)

The Food and Drug Administration (FDA) has approved for adult use many drugs that have been tested for adults but not for children. Yet clinicians often prescribe adult-approved drugs for children, a practice known as off-label prescribing, (1) because most drugs have not been tested in children,[1] and (2) because clinicians presume that the safety and effectiveness demonstrated with adults generally means that the drugs are also safe and effective for children. However, research shows, as described later in this report and in **Table 1**, that this is not always true. Children may need higher or lower doses than adults, may experience effects on their growth and development, and may not respond to drugs approved for adults.

Congress passed the Best Pharmaceuticals for Children Act (BPCA) of 2002 and the Pediatric Research Equity Act (PREA) of 2003 to encourage drug manufacturers to develop and label drugs for pediatric use.[2] BPCA offers manufacturers incentives to conduct pediatric-specific research. PREA requires certain pediatric use information in products' labeling.[3] The Food and Drug Administration Amendments Act of 2007 (FDAAA, P.L. 110-85)[4] reauthorized and strengthened the programs' authorizing legislation. The FDAAA authority for these two programs is set to end on October 1, 2012, unless Congress reauthorizes the efforts.

This report describes how and why Congress developed these initiatives. Specifically, the report

- describes why research on a drug's pharmacokinetics, safety, and effectiveness in children might be necessary;

---

[1] Estimates vary between 65%-85%, perhaps because analysts use different denominators (e.g., all drugs, or all drugs used by children). See, for example, Statement of Rear Admiral Sandra Lynn Kweder, M.D., Deputy Director, Office of New Drugs, Center for Drug Evaluation and Research, "Programs Affecting Safety and Innovation in Pediatric Therapies," before the Subcommittee on Health, House Committee on Energy and Commerce, May 22, 2007, http://www.fda.gov/NewsEvents/Testimony/ucm153848.htm.

[2] Best Pharmaceuticals for Children Act (BPCA) of 2002, P.L. 107-109. Pediatric Research Equity Act (PREA) of 2003, P.L. 108-155. For a list of acronyms used in this report, see **Appendix A**.

[3] In FDAAA, Congress also created a program to address medical devices used in children—the Pediatric Medical Device Safety and Improvement Act (PMDSIA) of 2007. See CRS Report RL32826, *The Medical Device Approval Process and Related Legislative Issues*, by Erin D. Williams.

[4] CRS Report RL34465, *FDA Amendments Act of 2007 (P.L. 110-85)*, by Erin D. Williams and Susan Thaul, presents detailed descriptions of these and other FDAAA provisions.

- presents why the marketplace has not provided sufficient incentives to manufacturers of drugs approved for adult use to study their effects in children;

- describes how BPCA provides extended market exclusivity in return for FDA-requested studies on pediatric use, and how PREA requires studies of drugs' safety and effectiveness when used by children (**Appendix B** analyzes how BPCA and PREA evolved from FDA's administrative earlier efforts);

- analyzes the impact BPCA and PREA have had on pediatric drug research; and

- discusses issues, some of which Congress considered leading up to FDAAA, that may form the basis of oversight and evaluative activities along with reauthorization efforts in 2012.

Understanding Drug Effects in Children

A drug cannot be marketed in the United States without FDA approval. A manufacturer's application to FDA must include an "Indication for Use" section that describes what the drug does as well as the clinical condition and population for which the manufacturer has done the testing and for which it seeks approval for sale.

To approve a drug, FDA must determine that the manufacturer has sufficiently demonstrated the drug's safety and effectiveness for the intended indication[5] and population specified in the application.[6] The Federal Food, Drug, and Cosmetic Act[7] (FFDCA) allows a manufacturer to promote or advertise a drug only for uses listed in the FDA-approved labeling—and the labeling may list only those claims for which FDA has reviewed and accepted safety and effectiveness evidence.

Once FDA approves a drug, a licensed physician may—except in highly regulated circumstances—prescribe it without restriction.[8] When a clinician prescribes a drug to an individual whose demographic or medical characteristics differ from those indicated in a drug's FDA-approved labeling, that is called *off-label use*, which is considered accepted medical practice.

Most prescriptions that physicians write for children fall into the category of off-label use. In these instances, because FDA has not been presented with data relating to the drugs' use in children, no labeling information is included to address indications, dosage, or warnings related to use in children. Faced with an ill child, a clinician must decide whether the drug might help. The

---

[5] FDA describes "indication" as a "[d]escription of use of drug in the treatment, prevention or diagnosis of a recognized disease or condition" (FDA, "Drug Development and Review Definitions," http://www.fda.gov/Drugs/DevelopmentApprovalProcess/HowDrugsareDevelopedandApproved/ApprovalApplications/InvestigationalNewDrugINDApplication/ucm176522.htm).

[6] For descriptions and discussions of the FDA procedure for approving new drugs, see CRS Report R41983, *How FDA Approves Drugs and Regulates Their Safety and Effectiveness*, by Susan Thaul, and FDA, "Development & Approval Process (Drugs)," http://www.fda.gov/Drugs/DevelopmentApprovalProcess/default.htm (see links).

[7] Federal Food, Drug, and Cosmetic Act (FFDCA), 21 U.S.C. §301 et seq.

[8] The FFDCA does not give FDA authority to regulate the practice of medicine; that responsibility rests with the states and medical professional associations.

doctor must also decide what dose and how often the drug should be taken, all to best balance the drug's intended effect with its anticipated and unanticipated side effects.

Such clinicians face an obstacle: children are not miniature adults.[9] At different ages, a body may handle a given amount of an administered drug differently, resulting in varying bioavailability. This occurs, in part, because the rate at which the body eliminates a drug (after which the drug is no longer present) varies, among other things, according to changes in the maturation and development of organs. Clearance (elimination from the body) can be quicker or slower in children, depending on the age of child, the organs involved, and body surface area.[10]

FDA scientists have described how drugs act differently in children, noting the kinds of unsatisfactory results that can occur when drugs are prescribed without the pediatric-specific information. These results include unnecessary exposure to ineffective drugs; ineffective dosing of an effective drug; overdosing of an effective drug; undefined unique pediatric adverse events; and effects on growth and behavior.[11] **Table 1** includes examples of drugs for which research has identified different responses between children and adults.

Table 1. Examples of Differences in Effectiveness, Dosing, and Adverse Events for Children Administered Adult-Tested, FDA-Approved Medications

Type of difference	Example of drug demonstrating this difference
Inability to demonstrate effectiveness	• some cancer drugs • buspirone (Buspar) for general anxiety disorder • some combination diabetes drugs
Children require higher doses than adults	• gabapentin (Neurontin) for seizures: in children less than 5 years old • fluvoxamine (Luvox) for obsessive compulsive disorder (OCD): in adolescents (12- to 17-year-olds) • benazepril (Lotensin) for hypertension
Children require lower doses than adults	• famotidine (Pepcid) for gastroesophageal reflux: in patients less than 3 months of age • fluvoxamine (Luvox) for OCD: in 8- to 11-year-old girls
Unique pediatric adverse events	• betamethasone (Diprolene AF, Lotrisone) for some dermatoses: not recommended in patients less than 12 years of age due to hypopituitary adrenal (HPA) axis suppression

---

[9] David A. Williams, Haiming Xu, and Jose A. Cancelas, "Children are not little adults: just ask their hematopoietic stem cells," *J Clin Invest.*, vol. 116, no. 10, October 2, 2006, pp. 2593-2596; and Stephen Ashwal (Editor), *The Founders of Child Neurology* (San Francisco: Norman Publishing, 1990).

[10] William Rodriguez, Office of New Drugs, FDA, "What We Learned from the Study of Drugs Under the Pediatric Initiatives," June 2006 presentation to the Institute of Medicine.

[11] Examples taken from a presentation by Dianne Murphy, Director, Office of Pediatric Therapeutics, Office of the Commissioner, FDA, "Impact of Pediatric Legislative Initiatives: USA," January 26, 2005, presentation to the European Forum for Good Clinical Practice; and Rodriguez, June 2006. Other sources include W. Rodriguez, A. Selen, D. Avant, C. Chaurasia, T. Crescenzi, G. Gieser, J. Di Giacinto, S.M. Huang, P. Lee, L. Mathis, D. Murphy, S. Murphy, R. Roberts, H.C. Sachs, S. Suarez, V. Tandon, and R.S. Uppoor, "Improving pediatric dosing through pediatric initiatives: what we have learned," *Pediatrics*, vol. 121, no. 3 (March 2008), pp. 530-539.

Type of difference	Example of drug demonstrating this difference
Effects on growth and development	• atomoxetine (Strattera) for attention deficit hyperactivity disorder
	• fluoxetine (Prozac) for depression and OCD
	• ribaviron/intron A (Rebetron) for chronic hepatitis C

Sources: Presentations by FDA scientists Dianne Murphy and William Rodriguez, 2006.

Such examples illustrate why some in Congress believe in the value of conducting studies in children of a drug's pharmacokinetics—the uptake, distribution, binding, elimination, and biotransformation rates within the body. Such studies can help determine whether children need larger or smaller doses than adults. They can also establish whether doses should differ among children of different ages. Clinicians could use pediatric-specific information in the FDA-approved labeling of drugs to help them decide which, if any, drug to use; in what amount; and by what route to administer the drug. Furthermore, well-designed, -conducted, and -disseminated studies in children can reveal information about potential adverse events, thereby allowing clinicians and patients' family members to make better decisions.

Why Manufacturers Have Not Tested Most Drugs in Children

Most drugs—65%-80%—have not been tested in children.[12] Manufacturers face many obstacles—economic, mechanical, ethical, and legal—that make them reluctant to conduct these tests.

The market for any individual drug's pediatric indications is generally small, resulting in a relative economic disincentive for manufacturers to commit resources to pediatric testing compared to drugs for adults. Because young children cannot swallow tablets, a manufacturer might have a mechanical hurdle in developing a different formulation (such as a liquid). The existing ethical and legal requirements encountered in recruiting adult participants for clinical trials may present even greater obstacles when researchers recruit children. Specifically, both the Department of Health and Human Services (HHS) and FDA have issued regulations concerning the protection of human subjects and direct particular attention to the inclusion and protection of vulnerable subjects such as children[13] (see textbox). Recruiting pediatric study subjects can be difficult because many parents do not want their children in experiments. Also, drug manufacturers face liability concerns that include not only injury but difficult-to-calculate lifetime compensation, made even more difficult regarding a child whose earning potential has not yet been established.

---

[12] See, for example, Statement of Rear Admiral Sandra Lynn Kweder, M.D., Deputy Director, Office of New Drugs, Center for Drug Evaluation and Research, "Programs Affecting Safety and Innovation in Pediatric Therapies," before the Subcommittee on Health, House Committee on Energy and Commerce, May 22, 2007, http://www.fda.gov/NewsEvents/Testimony/ucm153848.htm.

[13] HHS regulations are in 45 C.F.R. 46 Subpart D. FDA regulations are in 21 C.F.R. 50 Subpart D. Protection of children in research is discussed in CRS Report RL32909, *Federal Protection for Human Research Subjects An Analysis of the Common Rule and Its Interactions with FDA Regulations and the HIPAA Privacy Rule*, by Erin D. Williams. See, also, Institute of Medicine, *The Ethical Conduct of Clinical Research Involving Children*, Washington, D.C.: National Academies Press, 2004.

Congress has offered incentives to manufacturers for pediatric research for two main reasons. First, doctors prescribe drugs approved for adults despite insufficient pediatric-use studies. Second, enough Members of Congress have believed that, despite the difficulty in conducting such studies, children could be better served once the research was done.

FDA and the Protection of Children in Clinical Research

FDA has established certain principles and guidelines regarding child participation in research on FDA-regulated products. Regulations address the need to minimize risk, specifying considerations in different situations, such as when the research involves "greater than minimal risk but presenting the prospect of direct benefit to individual subjects" (21 C.F.R. 50.52); "greater than minimal risk and no prospect of direct benefit to individual subjects, but likely to yield generalizable knowledge about the subjects' disorder or condition" (21 C.F.R. 50.53); and "investigations not otherwise approvable that present an opportunity to understand, prevent, or alleviate a serious problem affecting the health or welfare of children" (21 C.F.R. 50.54).

In a 2008 presentation to the Pediatric Ethics Subcommittee of the FDA Pediatric Advisory Committee, pediatric ethicist Robert Nelson from the FDA Office of Pediatric Therapeutics described the "'nested' protections" of scientific necessity, parental permission, child assent, and appropriate balance of risk and benefit. Dr. Nelson presented the "principle of scientific necessity: Children should not be enrolled in a clinical investigation unless absolutely necessary to answer an important scientific question about the health and welfare of children."

Sources: 21 C.F.R. 50 Part D; and Robert M. Nelson, Pediatric Ethicist, FDA Office of Pediatric Therapeutics, "21 C.F.R. 50, Subpart D: Additional Safeguards for Children in Clinical Investigations of FDA-Regulated Products," presentation to the Pediatric Ethics Subcommittee of the FDA Pediatric Advisory Committee, June 9, 2008, http://www.fda.gov/ohrms/dockets/ac/08/slides/2008-4399s1-13%20%28Nelson%20Presentation%29.pdf.

BPCA and PREA:
Laws to Encourage Pediatric Drug Research

Although Congress has designed other laws (such as those affecting drug development, safety and effectiveness efforts, and general health care and consumer protection) to promote or protect the health of the entire population (including children), the Best Pharmaceuticals for Children Act and the Pediatric Research Equity Act (both sections of the Federal Food, Drug, and Cosmetic Act) authorize programs focused specifically on pediatric drug research. Congress first enacted BPCA and PREA in late 2002 and early 2003, respectively. In 2007, Congress authorized their continuation for another five years.[14]

When presenting information about the pediatric research provisions in law, more than one FDA representative has referred to "the carrot and the stick."[15] BPCA offers a carrot—extending market exclusivity in return for specific studies on pediatric use—and PREA provides a stick—requiring studies of a drug's safety and effectiveness when used by children. This section describes BPCA and PREA and compares them on key dimensions.

---

[14] CRS Report RL34465, *FDA Amendments Act of 2007 (P.L. 110-85)*, by Erin D. Williams and Susan Thaul, presents detailed tables comparing FDAAA 2007 with BPCA 2002 and PREA 2003, showing both changed and unchanged provisions.

[15] See, for example, FDA, "Should Your Child Be in a Clinical Trial?," January 13, 2010, http://www.fda.gov/ForConsumers/ConsumerUpdates/ucm048699.htm.

Best Pharmaceuticals for Children Act

Legislative History of BPCA

Congress enacted the current BPCA provisions in three separate pieces of legislation:

- the Better Pharmaceuticals for Children Act, enacted in the FDA Modernization Act of 1997 (FDAMA);
- the Best Pharmaceuticals for Children Act of 2002; and
- the Best Pharmaceuticals for Children Act of 2007, enacted in the FDA Amendments Act of 2007 (FDAAA).

See **Appendix B** for a discussion of the chronological development of BPCA and PREA.

This section covers the main provisions in the Best Pharmaceuticals for Children Act. The law addresses two circumstances: (1) when a drug is on-patent and a manufacturer might benefit from pediatric marketing exclusivity and (2) when a drug is off-patent or a manufacturer does not want additional marketing exclusivity.

Pediatric Marketing Exclusivity

For drugs that are under market exclusivity based on patents or other intact extensions,[16] FFDCA Section 505A (21 U.S.C. 355a) gives FDA the authority to offer manufacturers[17] an additional six-month period of marketing exclusivity in return for FDA-requested pediatric use studies (including preclinical studies) and reports.[18] Marketing exclusivity extends the time before which FDA grants marketing approval for a generic version of the drug. The provision applies to both new drugs and drugs already on the market (except a drug whose other exclusivity is set to expire in less than nine months).

Before FDA sends a manufacturer a written request for pediatric studies, the law requires that an internal review committee, composed of FDA employees with specified expertise, review the request. It also requires that the internal review committee, with the Secretary, track pediatric studies and labeling changes. In addition, it establishes a dispute resolution process, which must include referral to the agency's Pediatric Advisory Committee.

Exclusivity is granted only after (1) a manufacturer completes and reports on the studies that the Secretary had requested in writing, (2) the studies include appropriate formulations of the drug for each age group of interest, and (3) any appropriate labeling changes are approved—all within the agreed upon time frames. The law requires that the manufacturer propose pediatric labeling resulting from the studies. A manufacturer must provide supporting evidence when declining a request for studies on the grounds that developing appropriate pediatric formulations of the drug is not possible.

Applicants for pediatric marketing exclusivity must submit, along with the report of requested studies, all postmarket adverse event reports regarding that drug. The law also has several public notice requirements for the Secretary, including the following:

---

[16] The FFDCA authorizes marketing exclusivity in specified circumstances for pediatric studies, orphan drugs, new chemicals, patent challenges (FDA, "Frequently Asked Questions on Patents and Exclusivity," http://www.fda.gov/Drugs/DevelopmentApprovalProcess/ucm079031.htm).

[17] The laws refer to the *sponsor* of an application or the *holder* of an approved application. Because that entity is usually the product's manufacturer, this report uses the term *manufacturer* throughout.

[18] Authority under BPCA 2007 will sunset on October 1, 2012.

- notice of exclusivity decisions, along with copies of the written requests;

- public identification of any drug with a developed pediatric formulation that studies had shown were safe and effective for children that an applicant has not brought to market within one year;

- that, for a product studied under this section, the labeling include study results (if they do or do not indicate safety and effectiveness, or if they are inconclusive) and the Secretary's determination;

- dissemination of labeling change information to health care providers; and

- reporting on the review of all adverse event reports and recommendations to the Secretary on actions in response.

Extended marketing exclusivity may be an attractive incentive to a manufacturer with a product that is being sold under patent or other types of exclusivity protections.[19] It is not, however, relevant in two cases: (1) when products are no longer covered by patent or other marketing exclusivity agreements and (2) when a patent-holding manufacturer declines to conduct the FDA-requested study and, therefore, the exclusivity.

FDA-NIH Collaboration

To encourage pediatric research that extends beyond FDA's authority to influence manufacturers' research plans, BPCA includes provisions to encourage pediatric research in products that involve the National Institutes of Health (NIH).

Off-Patent Products

BPCA 2002 addressed the first group, which it described as "off-patent," by adding a new Section 409I (42 U.S.C. 284m) to the Public Health Service Act (PHSA). The new section established an off-patent research fund at NIH for these studies and authorized appropriations of $200 million for FY2002 and such sums as necessary for each of the five years until the provisions were set to sunset on October 1, 2007. Congress repeated the authorization of appropriations in the 2007 legislation.

BPCA 2002 originally required the Secretary, through the NIH director and in consultation with the FDA commissioner and pediatric research experts, to list approved drugs for which pediatric studies were needed and to assess their safety and effectiveness. The 2007 reauthorization changed the specifications from an annual list of approved *drugs* to a list, revised every three years, of priority *study needs in pediatric therapeutics*, including drugs or indications. The Secretary is to determine (in consultation with the internal committee) whether a continuing need for pediatric studies exists. If so, the Secretary must refer those drugs for inclusion on the list. When the Secretary determines that drugs without pediatric studies require pediatric information, the Secretary must determine whether funds are available through the Foundation for the NIH (FNIH). If yes, the law requires the Secretary to issue a grant to conduct such studies. If no, it

---

[19] The FFDCA authorizes marketing exclusivity in specified circumstances for pediatric studies, orphan drugs, new chemicals, patent challenges (FDA, "Frequently Asked Questions on Patents and Exclusivity," http://www.fda.gov/Drugs/DevelopmentApprovalProcess/ucm079031.htm).

requires the Secretary to refer the drug for inclusion on the list established under PHSA Section 409I.

Manufacturer-Declined Studies

For on-patent drugs whose manufacturers declined FDA's written requests for studies, BPCA 2002 amended the FFDCA Section 505A to allow their referral by FDA to FNIH for pediatric studies, creating a second avenue of FDA-NIH collaboration.

The law requires the Secretary, after deciding that an on-patent drug requires pediatric study, to determine whether FNIH has sufficient money to fund a grant or contract for such studies. If it does, the Secretary must refer that study to FNIH and FNIH must fund it. If FNIH has insufficient funds, the Secretary may require the manufacturer to conduct a pediatric assessment under PREA (described in the Pediatric Research Equity Act section). If the Secretary does not require the study, the Secretary must notify the public of that decision and the reasons for it.

Other Provisions

BPCA 2002 also established an FDA Office of Pediatric Therapeutics, defined pediatric age groups to include neonates, and gave priority status to pediatric supplemental applications. BPCA 2007 includes requirements for the Secretary. It expanded the Secretary's authority and, in some cases, requires action. For example, the Secretary must publish within 30 days any determination regarding market exclusivity and must include a copy of the written request that specified what studies were necessary. The Secretary must also publicly identify any drug with a developed pediatric formulation that studies have demonstrated to be safe and effective for children if its manufacturer has not introduced the pediatric formulation onto the market within one year.

BPCA 2002 also required two outside reports. First, it required a report from the Comptroller General, in consultation with the HHS Secretary, on the effectiveness of the pediatric exclusivity program "in ensuring that medicines used by children are tested and properly labeled." By law, the report was to cover specified items such as the extent of testing, exclusivity determinations, labeling changes, and the economic impact of the program. GAO released its report in March 2007.[20] BPCA 2007 requires another report that GAO released in May 2011.[21]

---

[20] In March 2007, the Government Accountability Office (GAO) issued a report that the BPCA legislation had required (GAO, *Pediatric Drug Research Studies Conducted under Best Pharmaceuticals for Children Act*, Report to Congressional Committees, GAO-07-557, March 2007). Noting that most of the exclusivity-associated studies resulted in labeling changes, GAO calculated the time that elapsed before those changes were completed. The entire process— from initial data submission, through FDA review and frequent requests for additional data, to follow-up submissions and reviews—took an average of nine months. One-third of the drugs' labeling changing took less than three months, whereas the labeling change for one drug took almost three years. The GAO report identified three main categories of labeling change: to inform of ineffective drugs, dosing that was too high or too low, and newly identified adverse events. It juxtaposed those findings with the statement that children take many of these drugs for common, serious, or life-threatening conditions.

[21] BPCA 2007 (FDAAA) directed that GAO submit a report by January 1, 2011. GAO briefed the committees on its findings on December 15, 2010, and later submitted its report (GAO, *Pediatric Research Products Studied under Two Related Laws, but Improved Tracking Needed by FDA*, Report to Congressional Committees, GAO-11-457, May 2011).

Second, BPCA 2002 directed the HHS Secretary to contract with the Institute of Medicine (IOM) for a review of regulations, federally prepared or supported reports, and federally supported evidence-based research, all relating to research involving children.[22] The IOM report to Congress was to include recommendations on best practices relating to research involving children. IOM released its report in 2004. BPCA 2007 requires another IOM report.[23]

Pediatric Research Equity Act

Legislative History of PREA

Congress enacted the current PREA provisions in two separate pieces of legislation:

- the Pediatric Research Equity Act of 2003, essentially codifying a rule FDA promulgated in 1997; and
- the Pediatric Research Equity Act of 2007, enacted in the FDA Amendments Act.

See **Appendix B** for a discussion of the chronological development of BPCA and PREA.

After passing BPCA, Congress acted to provide statutory authority for actions FDA had been trying to achieve through regulation. (**Appendix B** provides a brief history of those attempts.) The goal was to have pediatric-appropriate labeling for all FDA-approved drug products. The Pediatric Research Equity Act of 2003 (PREA, P.L. 108-155) added to the FFDCA a new Section 505B (21 U.S.C. 355c): Research into Pediatric Uses for Drugs and Biological Products.[24] It includes requirements for both new applications and products already on the market.

New Applications

According to PREA, a manufacturer must submit a pediatric assessment[25] whenever it submits an application to market a new active ingredient, new indication, new dosage form, new dosing regimen, or new route of administration. Congress mandated that the submission be adequate to assess the safety and effectiveness of the product for the claimed indications in all relevant pediatric subpopulations, and that it support dosing and administration for each pediatric subpopulation for which the product is safe and effective. If the disease course and drug effects were sufficiently similar for adults and children, the HHS Secretary is authorized to allow extrapolation from adult study data as evidence of pediatric effectiveness. The manufacturer must document the data used to support such extrapolation, typically supplementing the evidence with other data from children, such as pharmacokinetic studies.[26]

---

[22] See Institute of Medicine (IOM), *Ethical Conduct of Clinical Research Involving Children*, Committee on Clinical Research Involving Children (Washington, DC: National Academies Press, 2004), done with funding from NIH and FDA.

[23] BPCA 2007 (FDAAA) directed that the Secretary enter a contract with IOM by September 27, 2010. IOM has formed an ad hoc committee to consider "Pediatric Studies Conducted under BPCA and PREA"; it anticipates releasing a final report by February 2012.

[24] Unlike BPCA, which applied only to drugs, PREA applied both to drugs regulated under the FFDCA and to biological products (e.g., vaccines) regulated under the PHSA. In 2010, the Patient Protection and Affordable Care Act (ACA, P.L. 111-148) amended BPCA to add a pediatric market exclusivity provision for biological products.

[25] FFDCA ' 505B(a)(2)(A) describes the assessment as follows: "The assessments referred to in paragraph (1) shall contain data, gathered using appropriate formulations for each age group for which the assessment is required, that are adequate—(i) to assess the safety and effectiveness of the drug or the biological product for the claimed indications in all relevant pediatric subpopulations; and (ii) to support dosing and administration for each pediatric subpopulation for which the drug or the biological product is safe and effective."

[26] PREA 2007 authorized the Secretary to calculate pediatric effectiveness by extrapolating from adult data in certain (continued...)

The law specifies situations in which the Secretary might defer or waive the pediatric assessment requirement. For a deferral, an applicant must include a timeline for completion of studies. The Secretary must review each approved deferral annually, and applicants must submit documentation of study progress. All information from that review must promptly be made available to the public. In other situations, a waiver may be granted; for example, when the Secretary believes that doctors already know that a drug should never be used by children. In those cases, the law directs that the product's labeling include any waiver based on evidence that pediatric use would be unsafe or ineffective. If the Secretary waives the requirement to develop a pediatric formulation, the manufacturer must submit documentation detailing why a pediatric formulation could not be developed. The Secretary must promptly make available to the public all material submitted for granted waivers.

Products on the Market

PREA authorizes the Secretary to require the manufacturer of an approved drug or licensed biologic to submit a pediatric assessment. PREA 2002 and 2007 described the circumstances somewhat differently. The original provision applied to a drug used to treat a substantial number of pediatric patients for the labeled indications, and for which the *absence* of adequate labeling could pose *significant risks* to pediatric patients. PREA 2007, however, amended the provision so the Secretary could require a pediatric assessment of a drug for which the *presence* of adequate pediatric labeling "could confer a *benefit* on pediatric patients." PREA also applies when a drug might offer a meaningful therapeutic benefit over existing therapies for pediatric patients for one or more of the claimed indications.

Such situations could arise when the Secretary finds that a marketed product is being used by pediatric patients for indications labeled for adults, or that the product might provide children a meaningful therapeutic benefit over the available alternatives. The Secretary could require an assessment only after issuing a written request under FFDCA Section 505A (BPCA, pediatric exclusivity) or PHSA Section 409I (NIH funding mechanisms). Further, the manufacturer must not have agreed to conduct the assessment, and the Secretary had to have stated that the NIH funding programs either did or did not have enough funds to conduct that study.

If the manufacturer does not comply with the Secretary's request, the Secretary may consider the product misbranded. Because Congress wanted to protect adult access to a product under these circumstances, the law sets limits on FDA's enforcement options, precluding, for example, the withdrawal of approval or license to market.

(...continued)

circumstances. FDA cautions that "selection of an appropriate dose ... and the assessment of pediatric-specific safety should never be extrapolated" and that even efficacy extrapolation "requires an understanding of disease pathophysiology and the mechanism of therapeutic response" (Robert M. Nelson, Pediatric Ethicist, FDA Office of Pediatric Therapeutics, "21 C.F.R. 50, Subpart D: Additional Safeguards for Children in Clinical Investigations of FDA-Regulated Products," presentation to the Pediatric Ethics Subcommittee of the FDA Pediatric Advisory Committee, June 9, 2008, http://www.fda.gov/ohrms/dockets/ac/08/slides/2008-4399s1-13%20%28Nelson%20Presentation%29.pdf).

Other Provisions

Under PREA, the Secretary must

- establish an internal committee, composed of FDA employees with specified expertise, to participate in the review of pediatric plans and assessments, deferrals, and waivers;

- track assessments and labeling changes and make that information publicly accessible; and

- establish a dispute resolution procedure, which would allow the commissioner, after specified steps, to deem a drug to be misbranded if a manufacturer refused to make a requested labeling change. The law includes review and reporting requirements for adverse events, and requires reports from both the IOM and the GAO.

Seeing PREA and BPCA as complementary approaches to the same goal, Congress, in 2003 and again in 2007, linked PREA to BPCA (a discussion of this linkage appears later in the "Issues for Reauthorization of BPCA and PREA" section). Therefore, rather than specify a sunset date, Congress authorized PREA to continue only as long as BPCA was in effect.

Issues for Reauthorization of BPCA and PREA

BPCA sunsets on October 1, 2012, and current law authorizes PREA only as long as BPCA is in effect. As Congress considers a 2012 reauthorization, issues may emerge that were contentious in the 2007 reauthorization discussions. Those include the relationship between the two laws, cost, measuring the impact of the programs, labeling, and enforcement. This section reviews each.

Relationship Between BPCA and PREA

Although BPCA and PREA were developed separately, they are usually discussed—by policy analysts in FDA, Congress, and other interested organizations—in tandem. Their 2007 reauthorizations were paired in committee hearings and legislative vehicle (FDAAA) and Congress will likely consider them together in discussions of their 2012 reauthorizations. Now that BPCA and PREA have each been in effect for about a decade, it may be time to consider the rationale—whether planned or coincident—for two distinct approaches to encouraging pediatric drug research and product labeling.

Examining the Need for Pediatric Market Exclusivity

BPCA rewards pharmaceutical companies with extended market exclusivity for conducting studies on drugs for pediatric populations. In contrast, PREA requires pediatric studies. Legal analysts and some Members of Congress have speculated on this "carrot and stick" approach: Why Congress rewards the drug industry for something it requires the industry to do.

After reviewing the history of pediatric exclusivity when Congress was considering reauthorizing the FDAMA exclusivity provisions, one legal analyst wrote, in 2003:

If Congress had codified the FDA's power to require testing in all new and already marketed drugs, the notion of an incentive or reward for testing would appear ludicrous.[27]

In fact, Congress did exactly that: provided an incentive for something that is already a requirement. During the debate on PREA in 2003, Members of the Senate differed on this issue. In the Committee on Health, Education, Labor, and Pensions' report, Chair Judd Gregg [28] wrote, "The Pediatric Rule[29] was intended to work as a ... backstop to ... pediatric exclusivity." Disagreeing, Senator Clinton and others wrote in the report's "Additional Views" section:

> Neither the intent conveyed by FDA nor FDA's implementation of the [Pediatric] [R]ule supports the report's contention that the rule was intended to work as a "backstop" to pediatric exclusivity or to be employed only to fill the gaps in coverage left by the exclusivity.

Three years later, in its draft guidance on "How to Comply with the Pediatric Research Equity Act," FDA wrote that "[t]he Pediatric Rule was designed to work in conjunction with the pediatric exclusivity provisions of section 505A of the Act."[30] However, development of the Pediatric Rule pre-dated development of the exclusivity provisions.

The unclear relationship between voluntary studies for marketing exclusivity in BPCA and mandatory studies in PREA remained, continued by FDAAA 2007. At some point Congress may want to resolve this apparent paradox.

If, however, Congress were to consider eliminating pediatric market exclusivity or to somehow combine BPCA and PREA provisions, it might need to realign what the provisions cover. A recent FDA committee report describes one such difference.[31] It noted that, because PREA "requires studies only in the specific indication or indications" addressed in the new drug application (NDA),[32] PREA assessments would not include potential uses of the drug that would be unique to a pediatric population and therefore not be noted as an adult indication. If, however, the manufacturer sought pediatric market exclusivity for that drug, the studies required under BPCA would cover all uses of the active drug component.

Examining the Need for Permanent PREA Authorization

Not every law contains a sunset provision. BPCA does, and, although Congress did not use the term, it structured PREA 2003 to cease if and when BPCA did, reflecting the majority approach

---

[27] Lauren Hammer Breslow, "The Best Pharmaceuticals for Children Act of 2002: The Rise of the Voluntary Incentive Structure and Congressional Refusal to Require Pediatric Testing," *Harvard Journal on Legislation*, vol. 40, 2003, pp. 133-191.

[28] S.Rept. 108-84, to accompany S. 650, the Pediatric Research Equity Act of 2003, June 27, 2003.

[29] PREA effectively codified the FDA-promulgated Pediatric Rule; see **Appendix B** for additional detail.

[30] FDA "DRAFT Guidance for Industry: How to Comply with the Pediatric Research Equity Act," Center for Drug Evaluation and Research (CDER) and Center for Biologics Evaluation and Research (CBER), September 2005. http://www.fda.gov/downloads/Drugs/GuidanceComplianceRegulatoryInformation/Guidances/ucm079756.pdf.

[31] FDA Pediatric Review Committee (PeRC), "Retrospective Review of Information Submitted and Actions Taken in Response to PREA 2003," January 14, 2010, http://www.fda.gov/downloads/Drugs/DevelopmentApprovalProcess/DevelopmentResources/UCM197636.pdf.

[32] For a description of the drug approval process, see CRS Report R41983, *How FDA Approves Drugs and Regulates Their Safety and Effectiveness*, by Susan Thaul.

discussed regarding "Relationship Between BPCA and PREA" above—that these are coordinated programs. Therefore, both BPCA and PREA are now set to end on October 1, 2012. By including an end date or another indication of a predetermined termination date, Congress provides "an 'action-forcing' mechanism, carrying the ultimate threat of termination, and a framework ... for the systematic review and evaluation of past performance."[33]

The sunset provision for BPCA's exclusivity incentive to manufacturers has not yet engendered congressional debate. However, during PREA consideration in 2003, some Members had objected, unsuccessfully, to linking PREA's safety and effectiveness assessment and resulting pediatric labeling to the BPCA sunset. By the committee markups of PREA in 2007, some Members advocated making the mandatory pediatric assessments permanent. If Congress intended the PREA sunset to trigger regular evaluation of the law's usefulness, other legislative approaches may achieve that result more directly, such as by requiring periodic evaluations.

If, however, the intent was to test the idea of requiring pediatric assessments, the years between PREA 2003 and consideration of PREA in 2007 had provided four years of evidence. The House-passed bill for PREA 2007 would have eliminated PREA's link to the BPCA sunset provision; the Senate-passed bill continued it.[34] The enacted bill included the linkage written in the 2003 legislation. As it approaches the 2012 reauthorization of these pediatric research provisions and with another five years of evidence, Congress may wish to evaluate the usefulness and effect of that link before it decides whether to continue it.

Costs and Benefits of Pediatric Marketing Exclusivity

In assessing the value of BPCA's offering of pediatric market exclusivity, it may be useful to identify the intended and unintended effects—both positive and negative—of its implementation. When FDA grants a manufacturer a six-month exclusivity, who might benefit and who might be harmed? Congress could consider the cost implications as it sets policy in the reauthorization.[35]

The manufacturer. The manufacturer holding pediatric exclusivity incurs the research and development expenses related to the FDA-requested pediatric studies. It then enjoys six months of sales without a competitor product and a potentially lucrative head start on future sales.

Some researchers have examined the *financial* costs and benefits faced by manufacturers that receive pediatric exclusivity. One 2007 study[36] calculated the net economic benefit (costs minus

---

[33] CRS Report RS21210, *Sunset Review A Brief Introduction*, by Virginia A. McMurtry.

[34] Not all Senate committee members agreed. See, for example, Senator Clinton's comments at the Senate Committee on Health, Education, Labor, and Pensions hearing, "Ensuring Safe Medicines and Medical Devices for Children," March 27, 2007, at http://www.cq.com/?display.do?dockey=/?cqonline/?prod/?data/?docs/?html/?transcripts/?congressional/?110/?congressionaltranscripts110-000002481833.html@committees&metapub=CQ-CONGTRANSCRIPTS&searchIndex=0&seqNum=13; and S.Rept. 108-84, Additional Views.

[35] For example, although the BPCA reauthorization in 2007 continued the six-month exclusivity, the Senate bills under consideration at the time (S. 1082 and S. 1156 in the 110th Congress) would have limited the period of exclusivity for a drug to three months if its manufacturer/sponsor had more than $1 billion in annual gross U.S. sales for all its products with the same active ingredient. In future years, Congress might reexamine whether such limits are in the public interest.

[36] Jennifer S. Li, Eric L. Eisenstein, Henry G. Grabowski, et al., "Economic Return of Clinical Trials Performed Under the Pediatric Exclusivity Program," *Journal of the American Medical Association*, vol. 297, no. 5, February 7, 2007, pp. 480-488.

benefits, after estimating and adjusting for other factors) to a manufacturer that, in 2002-2004, responded to an FDA request for pediatric studies and received pediatric exclusivity. The median net economic benefit of six-month exclusivity was $134.3 million. The study found a large range, from a net loss of $9 million to a net benefit of over half a billion dollars.[37]

Other manufacturers. Manufacturers that do not hold the exclusivity must wait six months, during which time they cannot launch competing products. After that, however, they may be able to market generic versions of a drug that has been assessed for pediatric use and has had six months' experience in the public's awareness.

Government. Nonfinancial benefits to government include its progress in protecting children's health. Financial costs to the government include administrative and regulatory expenses. Because the government also pays for drugs, both directly and indirectly, it must pay the higher price that exclusivity allows by deferring the availability of lower-priced generics for six months.[38] The improved pediatric information, however, may yield future financial savings by avoiding ineffective and unsafe uses.

Private insurers. Private payers also face similar financial costs and benefits as public payers, without the regulatory costs of administering the program.

Children and their families. If the six-month exclusivity incentives effectively encourage manufacturers to study their drugs in children, some children may incur risks as study subjects; conversely, they and others might benefit from more appropriate use of drugs, including accurate dosing.

Labeling

Pediatric studies can produce valuable information about safety, effectiveness, dosing, and side effects when a child takes a medication. Such information benefits children only when it reaches clinicians and others who care for children (including parents). BPCA 2002, PREA 2003, and their 2007 reauthorizations, therefore, included labeling provisions to make the information available. As Congress drafts language to continue BPCA and PREA, it could address whether FDA has adequate tools with which to assess, encourage, require, and enforce the development and dissemination of the information clinicians could use to reach better treatment decisions. Before examining some specific questions for congressional consideration, this report reviews the current requirements for pediatric labeling.

Current Pediatric Labeling Requirements

FDA now requires, by law, pediatric usage information labeling in the following three sets of circumstances:

---

[37] An indepth examination of the financial effects of pediatric exclusivity is beyond the scope of this report.

[38] For example, a University of Utah research group examined the effect of the six-month pediatric market exclusivity on costs incurred by the Utah Medicaid program for three classes of drugs. Their extrapolation of Utah's $2.2 million extra cost led to a national Medicaid estimate of $430 million for those three drug classes over an 18-month period. (Carrie McAdam-Marx, Megan L. Evans, Robert Ward, Benjamin Campbell, Diana Brixner, Joanne Lafleur, Richard E. Nelson, Patent Extension Policy for Paediatric Indications, *Applied Health Economics and Health Policy*, vol. 9, no. 3, May 2011, p. 171).

1. the manufacturer has successfully applied (via an original new drug application [NDA] or a supplement) for approval to list a pediatric indication;[39]

2. the manufacturer has received pediatric exclusivity after conducting appropriate studies;[40] or

3. the manufacturer has submitted the safety and effectiveness findings from pediatric assessments required under PREA (added by the 2007 reauthorization).

By regulation, FDA requires pediatric-specific labeling in the following circumstances:[41]

(B) If there is a specific pediatric indication different from those approved for adults that is supported by adequate and well-controlled studies in the pediatric population, …

(C) If there are specific statements on pediatric use of the drug for an indication also approved for adults that are based on adequate and well-controlled studies in the pediatric population, …

(D)(1) When a drug is approved for pediatric use based on adequate and well-controlled studies in adults with other information supporting pediatric use, …

(E) If the requirements for a finding of substantial evidence to support a pediatric indication or a pediatric use statement have not been met for a particular pediatric population, …

(F) If the requirements for a finding of substantial evidence to support a pediatric indication or a pediatric use statement have not been met for any pediatric population, …

(G) … FDA may permit use of an alternative statement if FDA determines that no statement described in those paragraphs is appropriate or relevant to the drug's labeling and that the alternative statement is accurate and appropriate.

(H) If the drug product contains one or more inactive ingredients that present an increased risk of toxic effects to neonates or other pediatric subgroups, …

The PREA and BPCA reauthorizations in 2007 added the third set of circumstances of required pediatric labeling. When the Secretary determines that a pediatric assessment or study does or does not demonstrate that the subject drug is safe and effective in pediatric populations or subpopulations, the Secretary must order the label to include information about those results and a statement of the Secretary's determination. That is true even if the study results were inconclusive.

If studies suggest that safety, effectiveness, or dosage reactions vary by age, condition to be treated, or patient circumstances, then detailed information could be included in the labeling.

---

[39] In the first case, the labeling includes pediatric use information only if FDA approved the pediatric indication. If FDA turned down or the manufacturer withdrew a request for a pediatric indication, pediatric use information appears nowhere in the product's labeling. In addition, the fact that the manufacturer had made an unsuccessful attempt—and the research findings that blocked approval—would be neither noted in the label nor made public in other ways.

[40] When it comes to exclusivity, the labeling rules are different. If the studies required for exclusivity support pediatric use or specific limits to pediatric use (different dosing or subgroups), that information would go in the labeling. The labeling would also make clear if the studies did not find the drug to be effective in children or if FDA waived the requirement to study because children should not or would not be given the drug.

[41] Material is abstracted from 21 C.F.R. 201.57(c)(9)(iv).

BPCA 2007 also strengthened the effect of labeling requirements by mandating the dissemination of certain safety and effectiveness information to health care providers and the public.

Although not included in the pediatric sections, another provision in FDAAA 2007 may yield benefits for pediatric labeling. Regarding television and radio direct-to-consumer (DTC) drug advertisements, the law required that major statements relating to side effects and contraindications be presented in a clear, conspicuous, and neutral manner. It further required that the Secretary establish standards for determining whether a major statement meets those criteria.[42] The fruits of such inquiry could be applied throughout FDA communication.

Finally, BPCA 2003 had required HHS to promulgate a rule within one year of enactment regarding the placement on all drug labels of a toll-free telephone number for reporting adverse events.[43] Because FDA had not yet finalized a proposed rule it had issued in 2004, BPCA 2007 required that it take effect on January 1, 2008.[44]

Questions for Congressional Consideration

Labeling is useful if its statements are clear and applicable to the decision at hand. The labeling must also, however, be available and read—at least by prescribing clinicians. While an improvement over no mention at all, a statement such as "effectiveness in pediatric patients has not been established" still deprives a clinician of available information. The statement does not distinguish among

- *studies in children found the drug to be ineffective;*
- *studies in children found the drug to be unsafe;*
- *studies in children were not conclusive regarding safety or effectiveness;* and
- *no studies had been conducted concerning pediatric use.*

With BPCA and PREA, Congress has acted to encourage more informative labeling and the research that would make that possible. Having observed a decade of experience with these requirements, Congress may want to ask follow-up questions to help determine whether the laws need amending. Have the dissemination provisions mandated by BPCA 2007 been adequate? Has FDA been able to enforce the labeling changes that the agency deems necessary based on results of pediatric studies under BPCA and PREA? Should Congress consider strengthening enforcement provisions in the reauthorization bill? Now that the law requires all labeling to require a toll-free number for reporting adverse events, might Congress want to explore how that is implemented and whether it has had any effect?

---

[42] FDA, 21 C.F.R. Part 202 [Docket No. FDA–2009–N–0582] "Direct-to-Consumer Prescription Drug Advertisements; Presentation of the Major Statement in Television and Radio Advertisements in a Clear, Conspicuous, and Neutral Manner; Proposed rule," *Federal Register*, vol. 75, no. 59, March 29, 2010, pp. 15376-15387.

[43] FDA collects reports of adverse events from consumers, clinicians, and manufacturers. CRS Report R41983, *How FDA Approves Drugs and Regulates Their Safety and Effectiveness*, by Susan Thaul, describes FDA's authority and activities regarding adverse event report collection, review, analysis, and subsequent agency action.

[44] FDA issued the final rule on October 28, 2008. Its effective date is November 28, 2008, and its compliance date is July 1, 2009 (FDA [21 C.F.R. Parts 201, 208, and 209], "Toll-Free Number for Reporting Adverse Events on Labeling for Human Drug Products; Final rule," *Federal Register*, vol. 73, no. 209, October 28, 2008, pp. 63886-63897). BPCA 2007 limited the rule's application to exclude certain drugs whose packaging already includes a toll-free number for consumers to report complaints to their manufacturers or distributors.

Measuring the Impact on Pediatric Drug Research

Have the pediatric research encouragement programs had an effect? Is more research done on pediatric safety and effectiveness? Is more detail on age-group pharmacodynamics and dosing added to labeling? In general, is more information available to clinicians that could help them make appropriate prescribing decisions?

BPCA and PREA have created a measurable change in the numbers of drugs with labeling that includes pediatric-specific information. Still, not all drugs used by children have labeling that addresses pediatric use. FDA approved more than 1,000 new drug and biologics license applications from the beginning of 2003 through 2009.[45] Yet, the PREA (and its predecessor Pediatric Rule) and BPCA statistics note 394 pediatric labeling changes since 1998.[46]

FDA, through BPCA, has granted pediatric exclusivity for pediatric studies for 178 drugs.[47] Those drugs make up 45% of the drugs for which FDA had sent written requests to manufacturers for pediatric studies. FDA did not grant exclusivity for 14 drugs for which manufacturers had submitted studies in response to requests, but manufacturers did not pursue exclusivity for most of the other drugs.

As described earlier, BPCA 2007 shifted the level at which NIH set pediatric research priorities. Rather than creating a drug-specific list, NIH creates a condition-specific list. Accordingly, NIH (coordinated by the Obstetric and Pediatric Pharmacology Branch of the National Institute of Child Health and Human Development [NICHD]) listed 34 "priority needs in pediatric therapeutics," basically medical conditions, and interventions for each. Of the 45 drugs mentioned, 5 were still covered by their manufacturers' patents. Also listed were a few non-drug interventions: drug delivery systems (for asthma, for nerve agent exposure), health literacy (for over-the-counter drug use), and devices used in dialysis (for chronic liver failure).[48] It may be interesting to see whether this shift in priorities from drugs to conditions affects the funding of specific research and ultimate availability of pediatric-specific drug labeling.

Since BPCA and PREA were reauthorized in FDAAA, several reports have examined how FDA has implemented their requirements. GAO and the FDA Pediatric Review Committee (PeRC) that FDAAA established have offered assessments and recommendations for improvement. Congress may be interested in exploring those findings and crafting those recommendations into possible amendments to current law.

---

[45] For more information, see FDA, "Drug and Biologic Approval Reports," http://www.fda.gov/Drugs/ DevelopmentApprovalProcess/HowDrugsareDevelopedandApproved/DrugandBiologicApprovalReports/default.htm.

[46] FDA, "Pediatric Labeling Changes through September 28, 2010," http://www.fda.gov/downloads/ScienceResearch/ SpecialTopics/PediatricTherapeuticsResearch/UCM221329.csv.

[47] The count is based on BPCA statistics through 2010 (FDA, "Drugs to Which FDA has Granted Pediatric Exclusivity for Pediatric Studies under Section 505A of the Federal Food, Drug, and Cosmetic Act," http://www.fda.gov/Drugs/ DevelopmentApprovalProcess/DevelopmentResources/ucm0500005.htm).

[48] National Institute of Child Health and Human Development, "Priority List of Needs in Pediatric Therapeutics for 2008-2009 as of September 1, 2009," http://bpca.nichd.nih.gov/about/process/upload/2009-Summary-091509-1-rev.pdf. NIH also pursues pediatric drug research outside of its role in BPCA and PREA. For example, in August 2010, NICHD announced a request for grant applications (RFA) to address not yet understood molecular and other mechanisms of known side effects in children of atypical antipsychotics, cardiovascular drugs, highly active antiretroviral therapies, and depro-medroxyprogesterone acetate (NIH, "Molecular Mechanisms of Adverse Metabolic Drug Effects in Children and Adolescents(R01)," Request for Applications (RFA) Number: RFA-HD-10-010, http://grants.nih.gov/grants/guide/rfa-files/RFA-HD-10-010 html).

In May 2011, GAO reported to Congress, as required by PREA 2007, a description of the effects of BPCA and PREA since their 2007 reauthorization.[49] Along with a description of the procedures required by the provisions, GAO notes an area in which FDA needs to improve data resources in order to better manage the programs. Although FDA can report the number of completed PREA assessments, it was unable to provide a count of applications subject to PREA. GAO points out that, without that information, it is difficult for FDA to manage its timetables and for others to assess PREA's effect. In describing concerns of stakeholders, GAO mentions "confusion about how to comply with PREA and BPCA due to a lack of current guidance from FDA" and difficulties in coordinating the differing content and timetables of U.S. and European Union pediatric study requirements.

As required by PREA 2007, FDA created an internal expert committee—the Pediatric Review Committee (PeRC)—that, among other things, conducted a retrospective review of assessments, waivers, and deferrals under PREA through September 2007.[50] The required PeRC report found that, although the pediatric assessments were "generally of good scientific quality," if FDA provided more detailed advice on what it wanted, the assessments could be more consistent and useful. In a related observation, PeRC noted that "where there is evidence of specific discussion and documentation of the studies need to fulfill the PREA requirements ..., the PREA assessments generally were of higher quality."

Inconsistency in decisions about waivers and deferrals were seen in the earlier years of PREA and the report noted that with the PREA 2007-required PeRC, a higher level of pediatric drug development expertise was now available to support all 17 review divisions, some of which had no pediatricians on staff.

PeRC recommended that plans for and conduct of pediatric studies should begin early in the process of NDA development. This would be useful, in particular, to "correct problems in consistency between pediatric assessments in response to a Written Request [for BPCA] and those only in response to the PREA requirement." In keeping with its concern over varied scope and quality of research designs, PeRC recommended that (1) FDA review divisions discuss plans in detail approaching what they would cover in a BPCA Written Request to "be better able to assess the scope of studies need to provide adequate data for dosing, safety, and efficacy for use in the appropriate pediatric populations;" and (2) FDA provide more extensive descriptions of PREA postmarketing study requirements in its approval letters.

PeRC recommended that when assessments come after an application is approved, FDA should ask the manufacturer to submit a labeling supplement as required by PREA 2007. Furthermore, finding that "[r]esults from pediatric assessments were not consistently incorporated into labeling," PeRC suggested that "[c]onsistency in placement and language may increase the ability of clinicians and patients/guardians to find information in the label" and recommended that FDA issue a pediatric labeling guidance.

---

[49] GAO, *Pediatric Research Products Studied under Two Related Laws, but Improved Tracking Needed by FDA*, Report to Congressional Committees, GAO-11-457, May 2011.

[50] FDA Pediatric Review Committee (PeRC), "Retrospective Review of Information Submitted and Actions Taken in Response to PREA 2003," January 14, 2010, http://www.fda.gov/downloads/Drugs/DevelopmentApprovalProcess/DevelopmentResources/UCM197636.pdf.

Enforcement

FDA's postmarket authority regarding pediatric drug use labeling has been limited. Congress had given FDA the authority to use its most powerful enforcement tool—deeming a product to be "misbranded" and thereby being able to pull it from the market—but has not given the agency authority to require less drastic actions, such as labeling changes. Of interest to Congress may be whether the current authority is appropriate and sufficient to ensure safety and, therefore, whether FDA should have a wider range of options.

Pulling from the market a drug that many consumers rely on could, according to some health care analysts, do more harm than good. In its report accompanying its PREA 2003 bill, the Senate committee noted its intent that the misbranding authority regarding pediatric use labeling not be the basis for criminal proceedings or withdrawal of approval, and only rarely result in seizure of the offending product.[51] The 2007 reauthorization continued this limitation on misbranding authority.

The FDAAA, which encompassed BPCA 2007 and PREA 2007, included a provision outside its pediatric-specific sections to create a new enforcement authority for FDA: civil monetary penalties. Framed in the context of giving FDA tools to create meaningful incentives for manufacturer compliance with a range of postmarket safety activities, the provision listed labeling within its scope. In 2007 Senate and House committee discussions of what maximum penalties to allow, proposed one-time penalties were as low as $15,000 and proposed upper levels ranged up to $50 million. The enacted bill (FDAAA) states that an applicant violating certain requirements regarding postmarket safety, studies or clinical trials, *or labeling* is subject to a civil monetary penalty of not more than $250,000 per violation, and not to exceed $1 million for all such violations adjudicated in a single proceeding. If a violation continues after the Secretary provides notice of such violation to the applicant, the Secretary may impose a civil penalty of $250,000 for the first 30 days, doubling for every subsequent 30-day period, up to $1 million for one 30-day period, and up to $10 million for all such violations adjudicated in a single proceeding. The Secretary must, in determining the amount of civil penalty, consider whether the manufacturer is attempting to correct the violation.

What options should FDA have if a manufacturer that has already received the six-month pediatric exclusivity then refuses or delays making an appropriate labeling change? For studies that result in labeling changes, when should FDA make study results available to the public? In considering whether to strengthen FDA's enforcement authority within the context of pediatric research and labeling, Congress can address manufacturers' actions at many points in the regulatory process, if and when, for example, FDA notes a manufacturer's reluctance to accept the agency's requested study scope, design, and timetable; that a study's completion is clearly lagging or overdue; that a manufacturer does not complete such a study; or does not release its results to FDA, peer-reviewed publications, or the public; or that procedures to incorporate pediatric study results into a drug's labeling have not proceeded appropriately.

---

[51] S.Rept. 108-84.

Concluding Comments

Congress has repeatedly acted to encourage research into the unique effects of FDA-regulated drugs on children—with both "carrots" of financial incentive and "sticks" of required action. It has also required that drug labeling reflect the findings of pediatric research, whether positive, negative, or inconclusive. And, most recently, it has given FDA broader authority to enforce these requirements.

With each step of legislative and regulatory action over the years, Congress and FDA have tried to balance often conflicting goals:

- drug development to address needs unique to children;

- tools to encourage drug manufacturers to test drugs for use in children, despite the expense, opportunity costs, and liability risk;

- protection of children as subjects of clinical research;

- public access to up-to-date and unbiased information on drug safety and effectiveness; and

- prioritizing agency activities in light of available resources.

Concerns remain, though, about many of the issues discussed during the 2007 reauthorizations—as well as issues presented in the last section of this report. Such issues may surface when reauthorizations are due in 2012 or in the broader context of congressional interest in drug safety and effectiveness.

Appendix A. Acronyms

BLA	Biologics License Application
BPCA	Best Pharmaceuticals for Children Act
C.F.R.	Code of Federal Regulations
DTC	direct-to-consumer (as in DTC advertising)
FDA	Food and Drug Administration
FDAAA	FDA Amendments Act of 2007
FDAMA	FDA Modernization Act
FFDCA	Federal Food, Drug, and Cosmetic Act
FNIH	Foundation for the National Institutes of Health
GAO	Government Accountability Office
HHS	Department of Health and Human Services
IOM	Institute of Medicine
NDA	New Drug Application
NICHD	National Institute of Child Health and Human Development
NIH	National Institutes of Health
PeRC	Pediatric Review Committee
PHSA	Pub ic Health Service Act
PREA	Pediatric Research Equity Act
U.S.C.	United States Code

Appendix B. Current Law Evolved from Earlier Attempts

Before BPCA 2002 and PREA 2003, FDA attempted to spur pediatric drug research through administrative action. **Table B-1** shows the administrative and statutory efforts to encourage pediatric drug research. The following discussion highlights selected FDA-specific rules and statutes that relate to discussions in this report.

Table B-1. Administrative and Statutory Efforts to Encourage Pediatric Drug Research

Year	Action
1977	FDA pediatric guidance on "General Considerations for the Clinical Evaluation of Drugs in Infants and Children"[a]
1979[b]	FDA rule on *Pediatric Use* subsection of product package insert: *Precautions* section [21 C.F.R. 201.57] (in 44 Fed. Reg. 37434)
1994[b]	FDA rule revised
1996	FDA guidance on "Content and Format of Pediatric Use Section"[c]
1997[b]	Food and Drug Administration Modernization Act (FDAMA, P.L. 105-115), included the Better Pharmaceuticals for Children Act
1998[b]	FDA Pediatric Rule finalized (effective 1999; invalidated by a federal court in 2002)
2001	Adaptation of HHS Subpart D (pediatric) regulations [45 C.F.R. 46 Subpart D] to FDA-regulated research [21 C.F.R. 50 Subpart D]
2002	Best Pharmaceuticals for Children Act (BPCA, P.L. 107-109)
2003	Pediatric Research Equity Act (PREA, P.L. 108-155)
2007	FDA Amendments Act of 2007 (FDAAA, P.L. 110-85) reauthorized BPCA and PREA and enacted the Pediatric Medical Device Safety and Improvement Act

Source: CRS adapted and expanded material from Steven Hirschfeld, Division of Oncology Drug Products & Division of Pediatric Drug Development, Center for Drug Evaluation and Research (CDER), FDA, "History of Pediatric Labeling," presentation to the Pediatric Oncology Subcommittee of the Oncologic Drugs Advisory Committee, March 4, 2003, at http://www.fda.gov/?ohrms/?dockets/?ac/?03/?slides/?3927SI_01_Hirshfeld%20.ppt.

a. FDA, "Guidance for Industry: General Considerations for the Clinical Evaluation of Drugs in Infants and Children," September 2007, http://www.fda.gov/downloads/Drugs/GuidanceComplianceRegulatory Information/Guidances/ucm071687.pdf.

b. Discussed in Appendix text.

c. FDA, "Guidance for Industry: The Content and Format for Pediatric Use Supplements," May 1996, http://www.fda.gov/downloads/Drugs/GuidanceComplianceRegulatoryInformation/Guidances/ucm071957.pdf.

Rule on Drug Labeling: 1979

In a 1979 rule on drug labeling (21 C.F.R. Part 201), FDA established a "Pediatric use" subsection.[52] The rule required that labeling include pediatric dosage information for a drug with

---

[52] Originally at 21 C.F.R. 201.57(f)(9), this material is now at 21 C.F.R. 201.57(c)(9)(iv).

a specific pediatric indication (approved use of the drug). It also required that statements regarding pediatric use for indications approved for adults be based on "substantial evidence derived from adequate and well-controlled studies" or that the labeling include the statement, "Safety and effectiveness in children have not been established."[53]

Despite the 1979 rule, most prescription drug labels continued to lack adequate pediatric use information. The requirement for adequate and well-controlled studies deterred many manufacturers who, apparently, did not understand that the rule included a waiver option.[54] FDA, therefore, issued another rule in 1994.

Revised Rule: 1994

The revised rule attempted to make clear that the "adequate and well-controlled studies" language did not require that manufacturers conduct clinical trials in children. The new rule described how FDA would determine whether the evidence was substantial and adequate. If, for example, clinicians would use the drug to treat a different condition in children than its FDA-approved use in adults, FDA would require trials in children. However, if the drug would be used in children for the same condition for which FDA had approved its use in adults, the labeling statement regarding effectiveness could be based on adult trials alone. In such instances, FDA might also require pediatric study-based data on pharmacokinetics or relevant safety measures. The 1994 rule continued the 1979 requirement that manufacturers include statements regarding uses for which there was no substantial evidence of safety and effectiveness. It added a requirement that labels include information about known specific hazards from the active or inactive ingredients.[55]

Food and Drug Administration Modernization Act of 1997

Three years later, Congress provided another approach to increasing pediatric labeling. FDAMA (P.L. 105-115), incorporating the provisions introduced as the Better Pharmaceuticals for Children Act, created a Section 505A (21 U.S.C. 355a) in the FFDCA: Pediatric Studies of Drugs. It provided drug manufacturers with an incentive to conduct pediatric use studies on their patented products. If a manufacturer completed a pediatric study according to FDA's written request, which included design, size, and other specifications, FDA would extend its market exclusivity for that product for six months.[56] The law required that the Secretary publish an

---

[53] FDA, "Labeling and Prescription Drug Advertising; Content and Format for Labeling for Human Prescription Drugs; Final rule," *Federal Register*, vol. 44, no. 124, June 26, 1979, pp. 37434-37467.

[54] FDA would waive the required pediatric assessment for a drug that "does not represent a meaningful therapeutic benefit over existing treatments for pediatric patients and is not likely to be used in a substantial number of pediatric patients;" or for which "necessary studies are impossible or highly impractical because the number of patients is so small or geographically dispersed; or "there is evidence strongly suggesting that the drug product would be ineffective or unsafe in all pediatric age groups." Partial waivers could apply for specific age groups (FDA, "DRAFT Guidance for Industry: Recommendations for Complying With the Pediatric Rule (21 C.F.R. 314.55(a) and 601.27(a))," Center for Drug Evaluation and Research (CDER) and Center for Biologics Evaluation and Research (CBER), November 2000, http://www.fda.gov/downloads/Drugs/GuidanceComplianceRegulatoryInformation/Guidances/ucm072034.pdf).

[55] FDA, "Specific Requirements on Content and Format of Labeling for Human Prescription Drugs; Revision of "Pediatric Use" Subsection In the Labeling; Final rule," *Federal Register*, vol. 59, no. 238, December 13, 1994, pp. 64240-64250.

[56] Although market exclusivity is a characteristic of patent benefit, the FDA-granted exclusivity is not a patent extension; rather, it means that, during the six-month period, FDA would not grant marketing approval to another identical product (usually a generic). For more discussion of pharmaceutical patents and marketing exclusivity, see, for (continued...)

---

annual list of FDA-approved drugs for which additional pediatric information might produce health benefits. FDAMA also required that the Secretary prepare a report examining whether the new law enhanced pediatric use information, whether the incentive was adequate, and what the program's economic impact was on taxpayers and consumers.

Pediatric Rule: Proposed 1997, Finalized 1998, Effective 1999-2002

Also in 1997, FDA issued a proposed regulation that came to be called the Pediatric Rule.[57] The Pediatric Rule mandated that manufacturers submit pediatric testing data at the time of all new drug applications to FDA. The rule went into effect in 1999, prompting a lawsuit against FDA by the Competitive Enterprise Institute and the Association of American Physicians and Surgeons. The plaintiffs claimed that the agency was acting outside its authority in considering off-label uses of approved drugs. In October 2002, a federal court declared the Pediatric Rule invalid, noting that its finding related not to the rule's policy value but to FDA's statutory authority in promulgating it:

> The Pediatric Rule may well be a better policy tool than the one enacted by Congress (which encourages testing for pediatric use, but does not require it).... It might reflect the most thoughtful, reasoned, balanced solution to a vexing public health problem. The issue here is not the Rule's wisdom.... The issue is the Rule's statutory authority, and it is this that the court finds wanting.[58]

Author Contact Information

Susan Thaul
Specialist in Drug Safety and Effectiveness
sthaul@crs.loc.gov, 7-0562

(...continued)

example, CRS Report RL33288, *Proprietary Rights in Pharmaceutical Innovation Issues at the Intersection of Patents and Marketing Exclusivities*, by John R. Thomas.

[57] FDA, "Regulations Requiring Manufacturers to Assess the Safety and Effectiveness of New Drugs and Biological Products in Pediatric Patients; Final rule," *Federal Register*, vol. 63, no. 231, December 2, 1998, pp. 66632-66672.

[58] U.S. District Judge Henry H. Kennedy Jr. quoted in Marc Kaufman, "Judge Rejects Drug Testing on Children; Ruling Finds FDA Overstepped Authority in Forcing Pediatric Studies," *Washington Post*, October 19, 2002, p. A9.